# OBESITY AMENDMENT

## HOW TO LOSE WEIGHT THE HEALTHY WAY

Joy Gabriel M.

# Table Of Contents

# Introduction

Obesity is characterized as the strange or unreasonable fat collection that presents a risk to well-being. A body mass index (BMI) over 25 is viewed as overweight, and more than 30 is obese. The issue has developed to plague extent, with more than 4 million individuals losing their lives every year because of being overweight or obese as of 2017.

Obesity keeps on filling in grown-ups and youngsters. From 1975 to 2016, the predominance of overweight or obese youngsters and youths matured 5-19 years expanded more than 4x from 4% to 18% internationally.

Obesity is one side of the double burden of unhealthiness, and today a more significant number of individuals are obese than underweight in each district except for sub-Saharan Africa and Asia. When considered an issue just in big league salary nations, overweight and obesity are presently definitely on the ascent in low and center-pay countries, especially in metropolitan settings. By far most overweight or obese kids live in agricultural nations, where the rates of increment have been over 30% higher than that of developed nations.

# Obesity

Obesity is an intricate infection including an exorbitant measure of muscle-to-fat ratio. Obesity isn't simply a corrective concern. A clinical issue builds the risk of several diseases and medical conditions, e.g, coronary illness, diabetes, hypertension, and certain malignant growths.

There are several justifications for why certain individuals experience issues getting fit. Typically, obesity results from acquired, physiological and ecological variables, joined with diet, physical work, and exercise decisions.

Fortunately, even unassuming weight reduction can prevent the medical issues related to obesity. A better eating regimen, more of physical activity can assist you with getting in shape. Doctor-prescribed drugs and weight reduction strategies are extra choices for treating obesity.

Body mass index (BMI) is an estimation that considers an individual's weight and level to quantify body size.

In grown-ups, obesity is characterized as having a BMI of 30.0 or more, as per the Center for Disease Control and Prevention (CDC).

Obesity is related to a higher gamble of serious infections, like type 2 diabetes, coronary illness, and disease.

Obesity is everywhere. The CDC gauges that 42.4 percent of Americans 20 years of age and more had obesity from 2017 to 2018.

Be that as it may, BMI isn't the most important. It has a few
restrictions as a measurement.

As indicated by the CDC: Factors like age, sex, nationality, can
impact the connection between BMI and muscle versus fat.
Additionally, BMI doesn't recognize an overabundance of fat,
muscle, or bone mass, nor does it give any sign of the conveyance of
fat among people.

Regardless of these restrictions, BMI keeps on being broadly
utilized as a method for estimating body size.

The accompanying classes are utilized for grown-ups who are up to
20 years of age:

BMI                        Class

18.5 or under          underweight
18.5 to <25.0           normal weight
25.0 to <30.0      overweight
30.0 to <35.0          class 1 obesity
35.0 to <40.0      class 2 obesity
40.0 or over           class 3 obesity

Body mass index (BMI) is generally utilized as a basic and solid
approach to seeing if an individual is a sound weight for their
height.

For most grown-ups, having a BMI of 18.5 to 24.9 means you're
viewed as a sound weight. An individual with a BMI of 25 to 29.9 is
viewed as overweight, and somebody with a BMI of 30 and above is
viewed as fat.

While BMI is a helpful estimation for a many people, it's not precise for everybody.

For instance, the typical BMI scores may not be exact if you're extremely solid since muscle can add additional kilos, bringing about a high BMI when you're not an undesirable weight. In such cases, your waist perimeter might be a superior aide.

What's viewed as a solid BMI is likewise impacted by your ethnic foundation. The scores referenced above by and large apply to individuals with a white foundation. If you have an ethnic minority foundation, the edge for being viewed as obese might be lower.

Figure out what your body mass index (BMI) is by utilizing our BMI-adding machine.

BMI ought not to be utilized to resolve whether a kid is a sound weight, because their bodies are as yet creating. Address your GP if you have any desire to see if your kid is overweight.

Visiting your GP

If you're overweight or obese, visit your GP for counsel about getting more fit securely and to see if you have an expanded gamble of medical issues.

Your GP might get some information about:

your way of life - especially your eating regimen and how much physical work you do; they'll likewise find out if you smoke and how much liquor you drink
any conceivable basic foundations for your obesity - for instance, assuming you're taking drugs or have an ailment that might add to weight gain

how do you feel about being overweight - for instance, assuming it causes you to feel discouraged
that you are so propelled to get in shape
your family ancestry - as weight and other medical issues, like diabetes, are many times more normal in families
As well as working out your BMI, your GP may likewise do tests to decide if you're at the expanded hazard of creating unexpected issues in light of your weight.

These could incorporate estimating your:

circulatory strain
glucose (sugar) and cholesterol levels in a blood test
abdomen outline (the distance around your waist)
Individuals with extremely huge waist - by and large, 94cm or more in men and 80cm or more in ladies - are bound to foster weight-related medical conditions.

Your GP may likewise consider your nationality since it can influence your risk of fostering specific circumstances. For instance, certain individuals of Asian, African, or African-Caribbean identity might be at an expanded chance of hypertension. Sound abdomen estimations can likewise be different for individuals from various ethnic foundations.

After your appraisal, you'll be offered an arrangement to talk about the outcomes in more detail, pose any inquiries that you have, and completely investigate the treatment choices accessible to you.

# Diagnosis

To diagnose obesity, your primary care physician will regularly play out a physical test and suggest a few tests.

These tests include:

Taking your well-being history

Your primary care physician might survey your weight history, weight reduction endeavors, physical work and exercise propensities, eating examples and hunger control, what different circumstances you've had, meds, feelings of anxiety, and different issues about your well-being. Your primary care physician may likewise survey your family's well-being history to check whether you might be inclined toward specific circumstances.

An overall physical test

This incorporates estimating your level; looking at imperative signs, for example, pulse, circulatory strain, and temperature; paying attention to your heart and lungs, and analyzing your waist region.

Working out your BMI

Your doctor will check your body mass index (BMI). A BMI of 30 and above is viewed as obese. Numbers higher than 30 increase health risks and much more. Your BMI ought to be checked something like once per year since it can assist with deciding your general well-being dangers and what medicines might be suitable.

Estimating your waist boundary

Fat put away around the waist, some of the time called stomach fat may additionally expand the risk of coronary illness and diabetes. Ladies with a waist perimeter of more than 35 inches (89 centimeters) and men with a waist perimeter of more than 40 inches (102 centimeters) may have more health risks than individuals with more modest waist perimeters. Like the BMI estimation, waist boundaries ought to be looked at no less than one time each year.

Checking for other medical issues

Assuming you have known medical conditions, your primary care physician will assess them. Your primary care physician will likewise check for other conceivable medical issues, for example, hypertension, elevated cholesterol, underactive thyroid, liver issues, and diabetes.

BMI is an unpleasant computation of an individual's weight corresponding to their height.

Other more exact proportions of muscle versus fat and muscle to fat ratio dissemination include:

skinfold thickness tests
screening tests, for example, ultrasounds, CT outputs, and X-ray examines
Your doctor may likewise arrange specific tests to assist with diagnosing obesity-related health risks. These may include:

blood tests to examine cholesterol and glucose levels

liver capability tests
a diabetes screening
thyroid tests
heart tests, e.g electrocardiogram (ECG or EKG)
An estimation of the fat around your waist is likewise a decent
indicator of your risk for obesity-related diseases.

# Causes Of Obesity

Family history and impacts

The qualities you acquire from your folks might influence how much muscle versus fat you store, and where that fat is disseminated. Hereditary qualities may likewise assume a part in how proficiently your body changes over food into energy, how your body directs your hunger, and how your body burns calories during exercise.

Obesity will in general spat families
That is not related to the qualities they share. Relatives likewise will generally have comparable eating and action propensities.

Way of life decisions

Bad eating regimen

An eating routine that is high in calories, ailing in fruits and vegetables, brimming with fast food, and weighed down with fatty refreshments and curiously large parcels adds to weight gain.

Fluid calories

Individuals can consume tons of calories without feeling full, particularly calories from liquor. Other unhealthy refreshments, like carbonated drinks, can contribute to weight gain.

Idleness

If you have a stationary way of life, you can without much of a stretch take in additional calories consistently more than you burn during exercise and routine day-to-day exercises. Taking a gander at PC, tablet, and telephone screens is an inactive movement. The quantity of hours spent in front of a screen is highly connected with weight gain.

Certain infections and meds

In certain individuals, obesity can be followed for a clinical reason, like Prader-Willi disorder, Cushing disorder, and different circumstances. Clinical issues, like joint pain, additionally can prompt diminished movement, which might bring about weight gain.

A few prescriptions can prompt weight gain on the off chance that you don't repay through diet or movement. These prescriptions incorporate a few antidepressants, diabetes meds, antipsychotic meds, steroids, and beta blockers.

Social and financial issues

Social and financial elements are connected to obesity. Keeping away from weight is troublesome if you don't have safe regions to walk or exercise. Also, you might not have been shown sound approaches to cooking, or you might not approach better food varieties. Likewise, individuals you invest energy with may impact your weight — you're bound to foster obesity assuming you have companions or family members with obesity.

Age

Weight gain can occur at whatever stage in life, even in kids. However, as you age, hormonal changes and a less dynamic way of life increase your risk of weight gain. What's more, how much muscle in your body will in general diminish with age. These progressions additionally lessen calorie needs and can make it harder to keep off overabundance weight. On the off chance that you don't deliberately control what you eat and turn out to be all the more truly dynamic as you age, you'll probably put on weight.

Different variables

Pregnancy

Weight gain is normal during pregnancy. A few ladies find this weight challenging to lose after the child is conceived. This weight gain might add to the improvement of obesity in ladies.

Stopping smoking

Stopping smoking is often connected with weight gain. Furthermore, for some purposes, it can prompt sufficient weight gain to qualify as obesity. Oftentimes, this occurs as individuals use food to adapt to smoking withdrawal. Over the long haul, notwithstanding, stopping smoking is as yet a more noteworthy advantage to your well-being than proceeding to smoke. Your primary care physician can assist you with preventing weight gain in the wake of stopping smoking.

Absence of rest

Not getting sufficient rest or getting excess of rest can cause changes in chemicals that increase cravings. You may likewise hunger for food sources high in calories and sugars, which can add to weight gain.

Stress

Numerous outside factors that influence mindset and prosperity
might add to obesity. Individuals frequently look for all the more
fatty food while encountering upsetting circumstances.


Microbiome

Your stomach microbes are influenced by what you eat and may
contribute to weight gain or difficulty getting fit.
Regardless of whether you have at least one of these risk factors, it
doesn't imply that you're bound to foster obesity. You can balance
most risk factors through diet, physical work and exercise, and
conduct changes.

Individuals with obesity are bound to foster various possibly serious
medical conditions, including:

Coronary illness and strokes

Weight makes you bound to have hypertension and unusual
cholesterol levels, which are risk factors for coronary illness and
strokes.

Type 2 diabetes

Weight can influence how the body utilizes insulin to control
glucose levels. This raises the gamble of insulin opposition and
diabetes.

Certain tumors

Obesity might expand the gamble of disease of the uterus, cervix, endometrium, ovary, breast, colon, rectum, throat, liver, gallbladder, pancreas, kidney, and prostate.

Stomach related issues

Obesity improves the probability of creating indigestion, gallbladder sickness, and liver issues.

Sleep apnea

Individuals with obesity are bound to have sleep apnea, a possible serious problem in which breathing frequently stops and starts when sleeping.

Osteoarthritis

Obesity expands the pressure put on weight-bearing joints, as well as advancing irritation inside the body. These elements might prompt entanglements like osteoarthritis.

Serious Coronavirus side effects

Weight expands the gamble of creating serious side effects assuming you become tainted with the infection that causes Covid sickness 2019 (Coronavirus). Individuals who have serious instances of Coronavirus might require therapy in intensive care units or even mechanical help to relax.

# Food And Diet

It's a well-known fact that how many calories individuals eat and drink straightforwardly affects their weight: Polish off the very number of calories that the body burns over the long haul, and weight stays stable. Consume more than the body burns, weight goes up. Less, weight goes down. Be that as it may, what might be told about the type of calories: Does it matter whether they come from explicit supplements fat, protein, or starch? Explicit food sources entire grains or potato chips? The Mediterranean eating routine? Also, shouldn't something be said about when or where individuals consume their calories: Does having breakfast make it simpler to control weight? Does eating at drive-through joints make it harder?

There's an adequate examination of food varieties and diet designs that safeguard against coronary illness, stroke, diabetes, and other persistent circumstances. Fortunately, a considerable lot of the food varieties that assist with preventing sickness likewise appear to assist with weight control. Food varieties like entire grains, vegetables, natural products, and nuts. Furthermore, a large number of the food varieties that increase illness risk----boss among them, refined grains and sweet beverages are likewise figured weight gain. Conventional insight expresses that since a calorie is a calorie, no matter what its source, the best guidance for weight control is essential to eat less and practice more. However arising research recommends that a few food varieties and eating examples might make it simpler to hold calories within proper limits, while others might make individuals bound to gorge.

Do Carbs, Protein, or Fat Matter?

At the point when individuals eat controlled and consume fewer calories in research facility studies, the level of calories from fat, protein, and starch doesn't appear to issue for weight reduction. In examinations where individuals can openly pick what they eat, there might be a few advantages to a higher protein, lower carb approach. For constant sickness avoidance, however, the quality and food wellsprings of these supplements matter more than their overall amount in the eating routine. What's more, the most recent exploration proposes that a similar eating routine quality message applies to weight control.

Dietary Fat

Low-fat eating regimens have for quite some time been promoted as the way to a solid weight and great well-being. In any case, the proof simply isn't there: Throughout recent years in the U.S., the level of calories from fat in individuals' weight control plans has gone down, however, obesity rates have soared. Clinical preliminaries have found that following a low-fat eating regimen doesn't make it any simpler to get in shape than following a moderate or high-fat eating regimen. Concentrate on volunteers who follow moderate or high-fat eating regimens losing the same amount of weight and in certain examinations, a little more, as the people who follow low-fat eating regimens. Concerning disease avoidance, low-fat weight control plans don't seem to offer any unique advantages.

A contributor to the issue with low-fat eating regimens is that they are in many cases high in carbs, particularly from quickly processed sources, like white bread and white rice.

Higher protein consumption of fewer calories appears to enjoy a few benefits for weight reduction, however more so in momentary preliminaries; in longer-term studies, high-protein appear to perform similarly well as different kinds of diets. High protein consumes fewer calories and will generally be low in carbs and high in fat, so far, separating the advantages of eating heaps of protein from those eating more fat or less carbohydrate is troublesome.

However, there are a couple of motivations behind why eating a higher level of calories from protein might assist with weight control:

More satiety

Individuals will generally feel more full, on fewer calories, after eating protein than they do in the wake of eating carbs or fat.

It takes more energy to process and store protein than other macronutrients, and this might assist people with increasing the energy they consume everyday.

Further developed body synthesis

Protein appears to help people hold tight to slender muscle during weight reduction, and this, as well, can assist with supporting the energy-consumed.

Higher protein and lower carb further develop blood lipid profiles and other metabolic markers, so they might assist with preventing coronary illness and diabetes. Yet, some high-protein food varieties are more grounded than others: High intake of red meat is related to an expanded gamble of coronary illness, diabetes, and colon cancer.

Supplanting red meat with nuts, beans, fish, or poultry appears to bring down the gamble of coronary illness and diabetes. Furthermore, this diet technique might assist with weight control, as well. Scientists followed the eating routine and way of life of 120,000 people for 20 years, seeing how little changes added to weight gain over the long run. Individuals who ate more red meat throughout the review put on more weight about a pound extra. Individuals who ate more nuts throughout the review put on less weight about a half pound less at regular intervals.

Carbs

Lower carb, higher protein diets might have some weight reduction benefits temporarily. However with regards to preventing weight gain and ongoing sickness, carb quality is significantly more significant than sugar amount.

Processed, refined grains and the food sources made with them white rice, white bread, white pasta, processed breakfast cereals, and so forth are rich in quickly processed carbs. Potatoes and sweet beverages are as well. The logical term for this is that they have a high glycemic file and glycemic weight. Such food sources cause quick and enraged expansions in glucose and insulin that, temporarily, can make hunger spike and can prompt gorging and over the long haul, increase the gamble of weight gain, diabetes, and coronary illness.

For instance, in the eating regimen and way of life study, individuals who expanded their utilization of French fries, potatoes and potato chips, sweet beverages, and refined grains put on more weight over the long haul an extra 3.4, 1.3, 1.0, and 0.6 pounds separately. Individuals who lessen their intake of these food sources put on less weight.

Explicit Food sources that Make It Simpler or Harder to Control Weight

There's developing proof that particular food decisions might assist with weight control. Fortunately a considerable lot of the food sources that are gainful for weight control likewise assist with preventing coronary illness, diabetes, and other ongoing sicknesses. Alternately, food varieties and beverages that add to weight gain, boss among them, refined grains and sweet beverages likewise add to persistent illness.

Whole Grains, Fruits, and Vegetables

Whole grains, whole wheat, earthy colored rice, grain, and such, particularly in their less-handled structures are processed more leisurely than refined grains. So they gradually affect glucose and insulin, which might assist with keeping hunger under control. The equivalent is valid for most vegetables and organic products. These "slow carb" food sources have plentiful advantages for illness avoidance, and there's additionally proof that they can assist with preventing weight gain.

The weight control proof is more grounded for whole grains than it is for leafy foods. Individuals who expanded their intake of whole grains, organic products (not fruit juice), and vegetables throughout the 20-year concentrated on putting on less weight 0.4, 0.5, and 0.2 pounds less separately.

The calories from whole grains, fruits  and vegetables don't vanish. Probable happening that when individuals increase their intake of these food sources, they cut back on calories from different food sources. Fiber might be liable for these food varieties' weight control benefits, since fiber eases back absorption, assisting with checking hunger. Fruits and vegetables are additionally high in water, which might help people to feel more full on fewer calories.

Nuts

Nuts pack a lot of calories into a little bundle and are high in fat, so they were once viewed as a "no" for weight watchers. For reasons unknown, investigations discover that eating nuts doesn't prompt weight gain and may rather assist with weight control, maybe because nuts are rich in protein and fiber, the two of which might assist people feel more full. Individuals who consistently eat nuts are less inclined to have respiratory failures or die from coronary illness than the people who seldom eat them, which is one more motivation to remember nuts for a sound eating regimen.

Dairy

The U.S. dairy industry has forcefully advanced the weight reduction advantages of milk and other dairy items, dependent generally upon discoveries from transient examinations it has supported. In any case, a new survey of almost 50 randomized preliminaries finds little proof that high dairy or calcium intake assist with weight reduction. Likewise, most long-haul follow-up examinations have not found that dairy or calcium safeguards against weight gain, and one concentrate in young people viewed high milk intake as related to expanded weight.

One special case is the new dietary and way of life change review, which found that individuals who expanded their yogurt consumption put on less weight; expansions in cheese and milk intake, nonetheless, didn't seem to advance weight reduction or gain. It's conceivable that the valuable micro-organisms in yogurt might impact weight control, however, more examination is required.

Sugared Refreshments

There's persuading proof that sweet beverages increase the gamble of weight gain, obesity, and diabetes: A deliberate survey and meta-investigation of 88 examinations found a clear relationship between soda consumption with expanded caloric intake and body weight. In youngsters and youths, a later meta-examination gauges that for 12 extra ounce servings of sweet drink polished off every day, weight file increases by 0.08 units. Another meta-examination finds that grown-ups who routinely drink sugared refreshments have a 26 percent higher gamble of developing type 2 diabetes than individuals who seldom drink sugared refreshments. Arising proof additionally proposes that high sweet drink consumption builds the gamble of coronary illness.

Like refined grains and potatoes, sweet refreshments are high in processed sugar. The research proposes that when that sugar is conveyed in a fluid structure, as opposed to a strong structure, it isn't as satisfying, and individuals don't eat less to make up for the additional calories.

These discoveries on sweet beverages are disturbing, considering that youngsters and grown-ups are drinking ever-bigger amounts of them: In the U.S., sugared refreshments made up around 4% of day-to-day calorie consumption during the 1970s, however by 2001, addressed around 9% of calories. The latest information finds that on some random day, a big part of Americans polish off some sort of sugared refreshment, 25% drink no less than 200 calories from sugared beverages and 5 percent polish off no less than 567 calories which could be compared to four jars of sweet pop.

Fortunately concentrates in youngsters and grown-ups have likewise demonstrated the way that scaling back sweet beverages can prompt weight reduction. Sweet beverages have turned into a significant objective for obesity counteraction endeavors.

Fruit Juice

It's essential to take note that fruit juices are not a preferred choice for weight control over sugared refreshments. Ounce for ounce, fruit juices, even those that are 100% fruit juice, with no additional sugar are as high in sugar and calories as sweet soft drinks. So it's nothing unexpected that a new review, which followed the eating routine and way of life of 120,000 people for 20 years, found that individuals who expanded their intake of fruit juice put on more weight over the long run than individuals who didn't. Pediatricians and general practitioners suggest that kids and grown-ups limit fruit juice intake to simply a little glass a day.

Liquor

Although most cocktails have a bigger number of calories per ounce than sugared refreshments, there's no obvious proof that moderate drinking adds to weight gain. While the new eating regimen and way of life change investigation discovered that individuals who expanded their liquor intake put on more weight after some time, the discoveries differed by type of liquor. In many past examinations, there was no distinction in weight gain after some time between light-to-direct consumers and non-drinkers, or the light-to-direct consumers put on less weight than non-drinkers.

Diet Examples, Portion Size

Individuals don't eat supplements or food varieties in confinement. They eat food that fall into a general eating example, and scientists have started investigating whether specific eating routines assist with weight control or add to weight gain. Portion sizes have additionally expanded emphatically throughout recent many years, so has the utilization of fast food. U.S. kids, for instance, devour a more prominent level of calories from fast food than they do from school food, and these patterns are likewise remembered to be supporters of the obesity pandemic.

Dietary Examples

Diets that highlight whole grains, fruits and vegetables, appear to safeguard against weight gain, though some dietary examples with more red meat, sugared drinks, desserts, refined carbs, or potatoes have been connected to obesity. The Western-style dietary example is additionally connected to the expanded hazard of coronary illness, diabetes, and other persistent circumstances.

Following a Mediterranean-style diet, factual to safeguard against ongoing infection has all the earmarks of being promising for weight control, as well. The conventional Mediterranean-style diet is higher in fat (around 40% of calories) than the common American eating regimen (34% of calories), yet the vast majority of the fat comes from olive oil and other plant sources. The eating regimen is additionally rich in natural products, vegetables, nuts, beans, and fish. A 2008 precise survey saw that as in the overwhelming majority of studies, individuals who followed a Mediterranean-style diet had a lower pace of obesity or more weight reduction.

Breakfast And Snacking

There is some proof that skipping breakfast builds the gamble of weight gain and obesity, however, the proof is more grounded in kids, particularly youngsters than it is in grown-ups. Meal frequency and snacking have expanded throughout recent years in the U.S. By and large, kids get 27% of their everyday calories from snacks, principally from pastries and sweet beverages, and progressively from tidbits and candy. Be that as it may, there have been clashing discoveries on the connection between meal frequency, eating, and weight control, and more exploration is required.

Portion Sizes

Since the 1970s, portion sizes have expanded for food eaten at home, in grown-ups and kids. Transient investigations show that when individuals are served bigger bits, they eat more. One review, for instance, gave moviegoers compartments of old popcorn in one or the other enormous or medium-sized cans; individuals announced that they could have done without the flavor of the popcorn and all things considered, the people who got huge holders ate around 30% more popcorn than the individuals who got medium-sized holders. Another review showed that individuals given bigger refreshments would in general drink altogether more, yet didn't diminish their resulting food utilization. An extra review further proof that when given bigger portion, individuals would in general eat more, with no reduction in later food consumption. There is an instinctive allure for the possibility that portion sizes increase obesity, however long haul-planned investigations would assist with reinforcing this speculation.

Fast Food

Fast food is known for its enormous parts, low costs, high acceptability, and high sugar content, and there's proof from concentrates on adolescents and grown-ups that regular fast food utilization adds to gorging and weight gain. The CARDIA study, for instance, followed 3,000 youthful grown-ups for quite a long time. Individuals who had higher fast food consumption levels toward the beginning of the review gauged a normal of around 13 pounds more than individuals who had the most minimal fast food intake levels.

They likewise had bigger waist perimeters and more prominent expansions in triglycerides, and double the chances of creating metabolic disorder. More exploration is expected to separate the impact of eating fast food from the impact on the local individuals' lives, or other individual qualities that might make individuals bound to eat fast food.

A Solid Eating Routine Can Hinder Weight Gain And Ongoing Illness

Weight gain in adulthood is in many cases progressive, about a pound a year excessively delayed of an addition for the vast majority to see, yet one that can add up, after some time, to a significant individual and general medical condition. There's rising proof that similar fortifying food decisions and diet patterns that help prevent coronary illness, diabetes, and other ongoing circumstances may likewise assist with preventing weight gain:

Pick negligibly processed, whole grains, fruits and vegetables, nuts, fortifying wellsprings of protein (fish, poultry, beans), and plant oils.

Limit sugared drinks, refined grains, potatoes, red and processed meats, and other exceptionally processed food varieties, like fast food.

However the commitment of anyone eating regimen change to weight control might be little, together, the progressions could amount to an extensive impact, over the long haul, and across the entire society. Since individuals' food decisions are molded by their environmental factors, legislatures should advance arrangements and ecological changes that make good food sources more open and abate the accessibility and showcasing of unhealthful food sources.

# Intermittent Fasting

Intermittent fasting is an eating plan that changes between fasting and eating on a standard timetable. Research shows that intermittent fasting is a method for dealing with your weight and preventing a few types of infection. Yet, how would you make it happen? Furthermore, is it safe?

What is irregular fasting?

Many weight control plans center around what to eat, however intermittent fasting is about when you eat.

With intermittent fasting, you just eat during a specific period. Fasting for a specific period every day or eating only once several days in a week can assist your body with burning fat.

How does intermittent fasting function?

There are a few distinct ways of doing intermittent fasting, yet they are completely founded on picking normal time spans to eat and snack. For example, you could take a stab at eating just during an eight-hour time frame every day and snack for the rest of the day. Or on the other hand, you could decide to eat just a single meal daily for two days per week. There are various intermittent fasting plans.

Night-time without food, the body depletes its sugar stores and starts consuming fat. This is metabolic exchange.

Intermittent fasting stands out from the ordinary eating routine for most Americans, who eat all through their waking hours. If somebody is eating three meals per day, and they're not working out, then every time they eat, they're running on those calories and not consuming their fat stores.

Intermittent fasting works by dragging out the period when your body has copied through the calories consumed during your last dinner and starts copying fat.

Intermittent Fasting Plans

It means a lot to check with your doctor before beginning intermittent fasting. When you receive their approval, the genuine practice is straightforward. You can pick a day-to-day approach, which limits day-to-day eating to one six-to eight-hour time span every day. For instance, you might decide to attempt 16/8 fasting: eating for eight hours and fasting for 16 hours. Many people find it simple to stay with this example over the long haul.

Another, known as the 5:2 methodology, includes eating consistently five days per week. For the remaining two days, you restrict yourself to one 500-600 calorie meal. A model would be assuming that you decided to eat regularly on each day of the week except for Mondays and Thursdays, which would be your one-meal days.

Longer periods without food, for example, 24, 36, 48, and 72-hour fasting periods, are not better for you and might be causing harm. Going excessively lengthy without eating could urge your body to begin putting away more fat because of starvation.

What might I at any point eat while intermittent fasting?

During the times when you're not eating, water and zero-calorie refreshments, for example, dark coffee and tea are allowed.

However, what I like about intermittent fasting is that it considers the scope of various food sources to be eaten and delighted in. We suggest that individuals should enjoy eating great and nutritious food. Eating with others and sharing the supper time experience adds fulfillment and supports general well-being.

Most nourishment specialists, view the Mediterranean eating regimen as a decent outline of what to eat, regardless of whether you're attempting intermittent fasting. You can barely turn out badly when you pick perplexing, raw carbs like whole grains, mixed greens, solid fats, and lean protein.

Intermittent fasting benefits

Research shows that intermittent fasting periods accomplish more than copy fat. When changes happen with this metabolic switch, it influences the body and mind.

Numerous things occur during intermittent fasting that can safeguard organs against constant infections like type 2 diabetes, coronary illness, age-related neurodegenerative problems, even fiery inside sickness, and numerous diseases.

Here are some intermittent fasting benefits research has uncovered up until this point:

Thinking and memory
Discovery found that intermittent fasting helps working memory in animals and verbal memory in grown-up people.

Heart wellbeing
Intermittent fasting also developed circulatory strain and sleeping pulses as well as other heart-related problems.

Diabetes
In animal studies, intermittent fasting prevents weight gain.

Furthermore, in six brief examinations, obese grown-up people shed pounds through intermittent fasting.

Tissue health
In animals, intermittent fasting decrease tissue harm during surgery and further developed results.

Is intermittent fasting safe?

Certain individuals take a stab at intermitting fasting for weight control and others utilize the strategy to address ongoing circumstances like high cholesterol or joint pain. In any case, intermittent fasting isn't a great fit for everybody.

Before you attempt intermittent fasting (or any eating regimen), you ought to check in with your primary care practitioner before starting anything. Certain individuals should avoid attempting intermittent fasting:

Kids and teenagers under age 18.
Ladies who are pregnant or breastfeeding.
Individuals with diabetes or glucose issues.
Those with a background marked by dietary problems.

Individuals not in these classifications who can do intermittent fasting securely can proceed with the routine endlessly. It tends to be a way of life change and one with benefits.

Remember that intermittent fasting might contrastingly affect various individuals. Converse with your doctor assuming you begin encountering surprising nervousness, cerebral pains, sickness, or different side effects after you start intermittent fasting.

# Risks

Being overweight and obese might raise your gamble for specific medical issues and might be connected to specific close-to-home and social issues.

Type 2 diabetes

Type 2 diabetes is an illness that happens when your blood sugar is excessively high. 8 out of 10 individuals with type 2 diabetes are obese. Over the long run, high blood glucose prompts issues, for example, coronary illness, stroke, kidney infection, eye issues, nerve harm, and other medical conditions.

Assuming you are in danger of type 2 diabetes, losing 5 to 7 percent of your body weight and getting normal physical work might prevent or postpone the beginning of type 2 diabetes.

Hypertension

Hypertension is a condition where blood moves through your veins with power more noteworthy than ordinary. Hypertension can strain your heart, harm veins, and raise your gamble of respiratory failure, stroke, kidney infection, and death.

Coronary illness

Coronary illness is used to indicate a few issues that might influence your heart. On the off chance that you have coronary illness, you might have a respiratory failure, cardiovascular breakdown, unexpected cardiovascular passing, angina NIH external connection, or an unusual heartbeat. Hypertension, strange degrees of blood fats, and high blood glucose levels might raise your gamble for coronary illness. Blood fats likewise called blood lipids, incorporate HDL cholesterol, LDL cholesterol, and fatty substances.

Losing 5 to 10 percent of your weight might bring down your risk factors for developing coronary illness. In a situation where you weigh 200 pounds, this means losing just 10 pounds. Weight reduction might further develop pulse, cholesterol levels, and the bloodstream.

Stroke

Stroke is a condition where the blood supply to your brain is unexpectedly removed, brought about by a blockage or the blasting of a vein in your cerebrum or neck. A stroke can harm brain tissue and make you unfit to talk or move portions of your body. Hypertension is the primary source of strokes.

Rest apnea

Rest apnea is a typical problem wherein you don't inhale consistently while sleeping. You might quit breathing by and large for brief timeframes. Untreated rest apnea might raise your gamble of other medical issues, like type 2 diabetes and coronary illness.

Metabolic condition

A metabolic disorder is a condition that puts you at risk of coronary illness, diabetes, and stroke. These circumstances are

hypertension
high blood glucose levels
high fatty substance levels in your blood

low degrees of HDL cholesterol (the "upside" cholesterol) in your blood

an excess of fat around your abdomen

Fatty liver sicknesses

Fatty liver illnesses are conditions in which fat develops in your liver. Fatty liver infections incorporate Non-Alcoholic Fatty Liver Disease (NAFLD) and Non-Alcoholic Steatohepatitis (NASH). Fatty liver diseases might prompt serious liver harm, cirrhosis, or much liver disappointment.

Osteoarthritis

Osteoarthritis is a typical, enduring medical condition that causes torment, enlarging, and diminished movement in your joints. Being overweight or having obesity might raise your gamble of getting osteoarthritis by coming down on your joints and ligament.

Gallbladder illnesses

Obesity might raise your gamble of getting gallbladder illnesses, like gallstones and cholecystitis. Uneven characters in substances that make up bile cause gallstones. Gallstones might frame assuming that bile contains a lot of cholesterol.

A few tumors

Malignant growth NIH external connection is an assortment of related infections. In a wide range of diseases, a portion of the body's cells starts to isolate ceaselessly and spread into encompassing tissues. Obesity might raise your gamble of fostering specific kinds of malignant growth NIH external connection.

Kidney infection

Kidney infection implies that your kidneys are harmed and can't channel blood like they ought to. Obesity raises the gamble of diabetes and hypertension, the most well-known reasons for kidney infection. Regardless of whether you have diabetes or hypertension, the weight itself might advance kidney illness and revive its encouragement.

Pregnancy issues

Obesity raises the gamble of medical conditions that might happen during pregnancy. Pregnant ladies who are overweight or fat might have a more noteworthy possibility of

creating gestational diabetes
having toxemia — hypertension during pregnancy, which can cause extreme medical conditions for mother and child whenever left untreated
requiring a cesarean section NIH external connection, or C-section, and, subsequently, taking more time to recuperate in the wake of conceiving an offspring
What profound and social issues are connected to overweight and obese?

Being overweight and obese is related to emotional well-being issues like gloom NIH external interface. Individuals who manage overweight and obesity may likewise be the subject of weight inclination and shame from others, including medical services suppliers. This can prompt sensations of dismissal, disgrace, or responsibility, further demolishing emotional well-being issues.

# Treatment

If you're obese, address your GP for exhortation about shedding pounds securely.

Your GP can prompt you about getting in shape securely by eating a solid, adjusted diet and doing normal physical work.

They can likewise tell you about other helpful administrations, for example,

neighborhood weight reduction gatherings - these could be given the NHS, or business administrations you might need to pay for
On the off chance that you have basic issues related to obesity, for example, polycystic ovary syndrome (PCOS), hypertension, diabetes, or sleep apnoea, your GP might suggest further tests or explicit treatment. At times, they might allude you to a trained professional.

Read more about how your GP can assist you with getting thinner.

Diet
There's no single decision that applies to everybody, except to get more fit at a protected and practical pace of 0.5 to 1kg per week, many people are encouraged to lessen their energy consumption by 600 calories per day.

For most men, this will mean consuming something like 1,900 calories per day, and for most ladies, something like 1,400 calories per day.

The most effective way to accomplish this is to trade undesirable and high-energy food decisions - like fast food, processed food, and sweet beverages (counting liquor) - for better decisions.

A sound eating regimen should comprise of:

a lot of leafy foods
a lot of potatoes, bread, rice, pasta, and other boring food sources (preferably you ought to pick wholegrain assortments)
a few milk and dairy food sources
moderate amount of meat, fish, eggs, beans, and other non-dairy wellsprings of protein
simple modest quantities of food and beverages that are high in fat and sugar
Attempt to stay away from food varieties containing high degrees of salt since they can raise your circulatory strain, which can be risky for individuals who are obese. Read a few hints for a lower-salt eating routine.

You'll likewise have to check calorie data for each kind of food and drink you polish off to ensure you don't go over your everyday cutoff.

A few eateries, bistros, and fast food outlets give calorie data per section, although it isn't obligatory to give this data. Be cautious while eating out because a few food sources can rapidly take you over the breaking point, like burgers, broiled chicken, and a few curries or Chinese dishes.

Diet projects and craze "eat less" carbs

Stay away from the trend of "eat less" that suggests harmful practices, like fasting (doing without nourishment for significant periods) or removing whole nutrition types. These type of diets don't work, can cause you to feel sick, and are not feasible because they don't show you long-haul good dieting propensities.

It is not necessarily the case that all business diet programs are risky. Many depend on sound clinical and logical standards and can function admirably for certain individuals.

A dependable eating routine program ought to:

instruct you about issues, for example, portion size, rolling out social improvements, and smart dieting
not be excessively prohibitive as far as the kind of food sources you can eat
be founded on accomplishing steady, feasible weight reduction instead of transient quick weight reduction, which is probably not going to endure
Exceptionally low-calorie eats less
A very low-calorie diet (VLCD) is where you consume under 800 calories every day.

These eating regimens can prompt quick weight reduction, yet they are not a reasonable or safe strategy for everybody, and they are not regularly suggested for overseeing obesity.

VLCDs are generally possibly suggested assuming you have an obesity-related complexity that would profit from quick weight reduction.

VLCDs shouldn't normally be followed for longer than 12 weeks all at once, and they ought to just be utilized under the management of a reasonably qualified medical care practitioner.

Address your GP first when you're thinking about this type of diet.

Work out

Reducing how many calories in your eating routine will assist you with getting in shape, yet keeping a solid weight requires physical work to consume energy.

As well as assisting you with keeping a solid weight, physical work likewise has more extensive medical advantages. For instance, it can help prevent and oversee more than 20 circumstances, for example, diminishing the gamble of type 2 diabetes by 40%.

Grown-ups ought to do at least 150 minutes of moderate-intensity per week

Moderate-intensity action is any movement that builds your heart and breathing rate, for example,

lively strolling
cycling
sporting swimming
walking
On the other hand, you could complete 75 minutes of enthusiastic force movement in seven days, or a blend of moderate and lively action.

During lively action, breathing is extremely hard, your heart beats quickly and you might not be able to hold a conversation.

Examples:

running

high-intensity aerobics

You ought to likewise do strength activities 2 days per week. This could be as a gym exercise. It's likewise important that you separate sitting (stationary) time by getting up and moving around.

Your GP, weight reduction counselor, or staff can assist you with making an arrangement fit to your very own requirements and conditions, with feasible and persuading objectives. Fire a little and develop slowly.

It's additionally critical to find exercises you appreciate and need to continue to do. Exercises with a social component or practicing with companions or family can assist with keeping you spurred. Make a beginning today - it's barely past the point of no return.

Read more about the physical work rules for grown-ups and the physical work rules for older grown-ups.

You might have to practice for longer, every day to prevent obesity. To prevent obesity, 45 minutes to 1 hour of moderate-intensity action a day is suggested. To abstain from recovering weight in the wake of being obese, you might have to do 60 to 90 minutes of exercise every day.

Other valuable methodologies

Proof has demonstrated the way that weight reduction can find lasting success assuming it includes different methodologies, close diet, and way of life changes. This could incorporate things like:

putting forth practical weight reduction objectives - assuming you're
obese, losing only 3% of your unique body weight can
fundamentally diminish your gamble of creating obesity-related
complexities
eating all the more leisurely and being aware of what and when
you're eating - for instance, not being occupied by staring at the
television
keeping away from circumstances where you realize you might be
enticed to gorge
including your loved ones with your weight reduction endeavors -
they can assist with pushing you
observing your headway - for instance, gauge yourself consistently
and make a note of your weight in a journal
Getting mental help from prepared medical care practitioner may
likewise assist you with having an impact on how you ponder food
and eating. Strategies like cognitive behavioral therapy (CBT) can
be helpful.

Staying away from weight recover foods

You must note that as you shed pounds your body needs less food
(calories), so following a couple of months, weight reduction eases
back and levels off, regardless of whether you keep on following an
eating routine.

On the off chance that you return to your past calorie intake
whenever you've shed pounds, you'll probably return the weight.
Expanding physical work to as long as an hour daily and proceeding
to watch what you eat may assist you with keeping the weight off.

Medication

Various kinds of anti-obesity medications have been tried in clinical preliminaries, yet the ones in particular that have ended up being protected and successful are orlistat and liraglutide.

Orlistat

You can utilize orlistat if a specialist or drug specialist believes it's the right medication for you. As a rule, orlistat is just accessible on remedy. The main item available without a prescription straightforwardly from drug stores is Alli, under the oversight of a drug specialist.

Orlistat works by hindering around 33% of the fat from the food you eat from being assimilated. The undigested fat isn't assimilated into your body and is dropped with your crap. This will assist you with trying not to put on weight, yet won't be guaranteed to make you get in shape.

You'll have to begin a fair eating regimen and exercise program before starting treatment with orlistat, and proceed with this program during treatment and after you quit taking orlistat.

When orlistat ought to be utilized

Orlistat will generally possibly be suggested if you've put forth a critical attempt to get thinner through diet, practice, or changing your way of life.

That being said, orlistat is possibly endorsed if you have:

A BMI of at least 28, and other weight-related conditions, for example, hypertension or type 2 diabetes
a BMI of at least 30
Orlistat isn't typically suggested for pregnant or breastfeeding ladies.

Before endorsing orlistat, your doctor will talk about the advantages and expected impediments with you, including any possible incidental effects.

Heed your primary care physician's guidance about how to take it and the guidelines that accompany your medication.

What amount of time is required

Treatment with orlistat ought to possibly last for 90 days assuming you've lost 5% of your body weight. It begins to influence how you digest fat in 1 to 2 days.

If you have not shed pounds in the wake of taking orlistat for a long time, being a successful treatment for you is impossible. Ask your doctor or drug specialist, as you might have to stop your treatment.

Orlistat and other medical issues

If you're taking medication for another serious ailment, for example, type 2 diabetes, hypertension, or kidney illness, changing the portion of your medicine might be important. Address your GP before beginning treatment with orlistat.

Assuming that you have type 2 diabetes, it might take you longer to get fit utilizing orlistat, so your objective weight reduction following 3 months might be marginally lower.

Results of orlistat

Normal results of orlistat include:

a sleek release from your rectum (you might have slick spots on your clothing)

flatulating (fart)

You're substantially less liable to get these secondary effects if you adhere to a low-fat eating routine.

If you're taking the oral preventative pill and you have serious loose bowels while taking orlistat, utilize an extra technique for contraception, like a condom. This is because your body may not assimilate the prophylactic pill assuming you have loose bowels, so it may not be powerful. Look at the pill bundle for exhortation.

Liraglutide

Liraglutide (likewise called Saxenda) is a weight reduction medication that works by causing you to feel more full and less ravenous. It's taken as an infusion one time each day. Your doctor will prescribe it to you in the best way possible.

You can typically possibly take liraglutide on the off chance that it's endorsed for you by an expert. A specialist could suggest that you take it if:

diet and exercise changes have not dealt with their own

orlistat has not worked or you can't take it

you would rather not have a weight reduction medical procedure

You'll have to go on with an eating regimen and exercise plan while taking liraglutide.

Before recommending liraglutide, your doctor will talk you through its advantages and restrictions, including any incidental effects you could get.

When liraglutide ought to be utilized

Liraglutide is reasonable for grown-ups matured up to 75. It isn't suggested if you're pregnant or breastfeeding or have specific ailments, like liver or kidney issues.

You'll possibly be endorsed liraglutide if these apply:

you have a BMI of at least 35, or you have a BMI of 32.5 or more and you're of South Asian, Chinese, Black African, or African-Caribbean origin.

you have non-diabetic hyperglycemia (high glucose).

you're at high risk of heart issues, for example, cardiovascular failures and strokes, since you have hypertension (hypertension).

What amount of time is required

You'll have a survey in the wake of taking liraglutide for quite a long time. You'll then, at that point, possibly continue taking it assuming you've lost no less than 5% of your body weight.

Surgery

Weight reduction surgery additionally called bariatric medical procedure, is most of the time used to treat seriously fat individuals.

Bariatric medical procedure is typically just accessible on the NHS to treat individuals with serious obesity who satisfy the following measures in general:

they have a BMI of at least 40, or somewhere in the range of 35 and 40, and one more serious medical issue that could be improved with weight reduction, for example, type 2 diabetes or hypertension
all fitting non-careful measures have been attempted, yet the individual hasn't accomplished or kept up with satisfactory, clinically useful weight reduction
the individual is adequately fit to have sedation and surgery
the individual has been getting or will get, serious administration as a feature of their treatment
the individual focuses on the requirement for long-haul follow-up

Bariatric medical procedures may likewise be considered as a potential therapy choice for individuals with a BMI of 30 to 35 who have as of late (over the most recent 10 years) been determined to have type 2 diabetes.

In uncommon cases, surgery might be suggested as the main therapy (rather than way-of-life therapies and prescription) if an individual's BMI is 50 or above.

Treating obesity in kids

Treating obesity in kids generally includes enhancements to eating less and expanding physical work utilizing conduct change procedures.

How many calories your kid ought to eat every day will rely upon their age and level. Your GP ought to have the option to prompt you about a suggested day as far as possible, and they may likewise have the option to allude you to your neighborhood family's sound way of life program.

Kids beyond 5 years old should get no less than an hour of fiery force practice a day, like running or playing football or netball. Stationary exercises, for example, staring at the TV and playing PC games, ought to be limited.

Read more about the physical work rules for kids.

Reference to an expert in treating youth obesity might be suggested if your youngster fosters an obesity-related difficulty, or if there's believed to be a hidden ailment causing obesity.

The utilization of orlistat in youngsters is just suggested in outstanding conditions, for example, if a kid is seriously obese and has an obesity-related entanglement.

Bariatric medical procedure isn't for the most part suggested for kids, yet might be considered for kids in uncommon conditions, assuming that they've accomplished, or almost accomplished physiological development.

9 798357 750594